Also by Barry Krakow
(co-author Joseph Neidhardt)

Conquering Bad Dreams & Nightmares
A Guide to Understanding, Interpretation and Cure

INSOMNIA CURES
Sleep Hygiene
Practice Makes Permanent

INSOMNIA CURES

Sleep Hygiene
Practice Makes Permanent

by

Barry Krakow, M.D.

THE NEW SLEEPY TIMES

Cover Photograph by Jessica Krakow

ISBN: 0-9715869-0-X

Library of Congress Control Number: 2001098304

To my darling Jessica

TABLE OF CONTENTS

ACKNOWLEDGMENTS

I want to thank Vicki Ahl, Fritz Eberle, Carol Jessop, Bruce Mann, and Dan Sperling for assisting me in the development of the book, editorial review, proof-reading, and preparation of the manuscript and cover.

PREFACE

I have personally experienced the misery and frustration of insomnia. My first episodes with insomnia were minor—I could not fall asleep before the first day of school for most of my childhood. That was it. But in my twenties and thirties, I noticed occasional difficulties falling asleep at night. This subsided in medical school and residency because I was so painfully sleep deprived that I could sleep anywhere and everywhere. In my late thirties and early forties, it returned again in mild form, and I simply made good use of my unslept hours by writing. In my mid-forties however I developed moderate and occasionally severe insomnia, ironically enough only a few years after I completed my formal training and board certification in sleep disorders medicine.

For the next five years, I tried everything short of sedatives to fix the problem, and in 1998 I discovered a cure for my insomnia. The cure that I discovered for myself, incidentally, is not the topic of this book, and that is so because there was *something* that I had to learn first and foremost to be able to accept and attempt the ultimate cure for my sleep disorder.

That *something* proved to be the principles and practice of sleep hygiene, which by studying closely and applying diligently to my problem led me to immediate improvements and eventually along a path of discovery that has almost completely eliminated my insomnia.

For more than a decade I have been instructing crime victims and other trauma survivors who suffer from some of the worst insomnia problems imaginable, and it always surprises me how much benefit they can attain through the principles and practice of sleep hygiene. Even so, let me reiterate, many of these individuals also suffered from other problems that affected their sleep, both mental and physical problems, and by addressing these aspects, some of them have also experienced a cure. However, as I learned for myself and they have learned as well, few of them could have progressed toward that cure until they first mastered and applied a sleep hygiene strategy.

Most people, although certainly not all, do need to crawl before they walk, and perhaps all need to walk before they run. Just so, sleep hygiene can help virtually every type of insomniac improve their sleeplessness, and most importantly, move them in a direction that will bring them closer to a full recovery of their normal sleep. For some people with mild or moderate insomnia, sleep hygiene may be a cure-all, although this is less likely for severe cases.

If you are an insomniac, for whatever reason and to whatever extent, there is a distinct possibility that a cure for your problem is attainable. And, in my personal and professional experience, as a first step towards that cure, I encourage you to closely examine and apply the principles of sleep hygiene.

Introduction

To understand why you may not be able to fall asleep or stay asleep is often a fairly easy knot to untangle. The more difficult part is learning how and when to apply the specific remedies that will reduce or eliminate your sleeplessness. For example, suppose you were to discover in the course of reading this book that one *cause* of your sleeplessness is that you engage in clock-watching at night to monitor how much sleep you are missing out on while lying awake in bed. Clock-watching is a remarkably common behavior engaged in by insomniacs, regardless of whether their insomnia is related to nightmares, depression, shift work, arthritic pains, other mental and physical disorders, or just about any other cause you might imagine. And for all these people suffering from insomnia, there is something on the order of a 95% chance that clock-watching is fueling or worsening their sleeplessness.

Notwithstanding the above, if I were to ask you to switch your clock so it faced the wall or to move the timepiece out of the bedroom entirely, it often turns out to be a case of "easier said than done." In other words, here's a BEHAVIOR (clock-watching) that is simple to define, which has been scientifically documented to be associated with insomnia. But, if I were to offer you a NEW BEHAVIOR (turn the clock face to the wall), which may prove to be a critically important step in recovering your normal sleep, your chances of an outright acceptance of this strategy are likely to be quite low, especially if you have suffered from insomnia for any appreciable length of time.

In my professional experience, this behavioral recommendation (avoid clock-watching) would be akin to telling an overweight person that all they really need to do is stop eating so much food. It may be as true as true can be that if you eat less, you'll lose weight, but so what, the real dilemma is learning the why and the how of not eating so much, and for many people that might take awhile to figure out.

This book avoids a simplistic behavioral approach, that is, I am more than willing to offer up the standard, quick-acting, and essential sleep hygiene solutions. However, at the same time, I will also provide you with a new way of thinking about the problem of insomnia and a new way of thinking about various sleep solutions so that you can apply this knowledge with greater confidence in treating your own sleeplessness.

If the dilemma you faced were analogous to crossing a river, which now seems uncrossable to you, this book will help you find the energy and motivation to build a boat or a bridge to meet the challenge.

We will accomplish this by recognizing that while all our sleep-negating BEHAVIORS are often easily spotted, it is our cognitions—our thoughts, ideas, attitudes and beliefs—about these behaviors that almost always have a stronger influence on our sleep problems. These cognitions will therefore ultimately hinder or help us in our quest to overcome insomnia. In fact, with respect to the BEHAVIORAL notions I've outlined above, it is actually the combination of COGNITIVE and BEHAVIORAL strategies that will prove the most effective in dealing with sleeplessness.

Thus, I can inform you, with considerable certainty, that many patients with insomnia do have difficulty in turning their clocks to face the wall when it is offered as a simple, quick fix. But, if we can add a COGNITIVE strategy to this NEW BEHAVIOR, I can tell you with equal certainty that the Sandman will soon be whispering in your ear.

1

IS YOUR BEDROOM THE ENEMY?

QUICK GUIDE

Problem: You arrive in the bedroom sleepy only to feel wide awake as soon as your head hits the pillow.

Cause: You've developed the habit of connecting your bedroom with mental alertness, which thwarts your natural ability to fall asleep.

Solution: Leave the bedroom and return once you feel sleepy again.

◆ ◆ ◆

You're tired, exhausted, ready to drop. It's three yawns past 11 o'clock and blessed sleep is just around the corner in your bedroom. You plop into bed, pull up the covers, roll over once, twice, settle down and then . . .

. . . unbelievably, you're wide awake!

This is one of the most classic forms of insomnia. At the moment of truth, it seems like you're about to fall asleep. Even before you land on the mattress, you can imagine nothing else but your head hitting the pillow followed by a quick visit from the Sandman.

Instead, you awaken, and more often than not, you spend another twenty, thirty and sometimes more than sixty minutes trying to get to sleep. Worse, you worry about how awful the next day will be. No matter how much you had hoped to accomplish, despite all your best plans, you now know you'll be dragging around much of the day warding off fatigue, exhaustion and sometimes a genuine desire to fall asleep.

To add insult to injury, you ask yourself "why does this happen to me? Why can't I do what so many other people seem to be able to do quite naturally — fall asleep and stay asleep?" There's almost a sense of guilt or blame for not getting the job done. It's as if sleep has become something you must "perform." In a real sense, anxiety performance occurs regularly at bedtime. This adds to your self-consciousness and aggravation about the sleeplessness, and in turn, makes the problem worse.

The good news about this type of insomnia is that it will almost always respond, in part, to the principles and practice of sleep hygiene.

Sleep hygiene encompasses many of the behaviors and habits in your daily life that affect your ability to sleep.

Overall, good sleep hygiene means creating an environment for yourself that promotes sound sleep. This environment includes physical things, like the type of mattress you might sleep on or the degree of light in your bedroom. It can include mental things such as learning to trust yourself to fall asleep. Most of all, proper sleep hygiene means learning how to establish a VERY STRONG AND

POSITIVE ASSOCIATION OR CONNECTION BETWEEN YOUR BEDROOM
AND GOOD SLEEP.

If you've experienced the aggravation of becoming alert
once you've entered your bedroom, then your **connection** between
the bed and sleep is no longer optimal. Instead, somewhere in your
mind and body, you have developed some nervousness about your
ability to sleep well. Therefore, when you enter the bedroom,
thoughts and feelings are triggered that eventually wake you up
instead of letting you doze off.

By using sleep hygiene principles, you can learn how to
trust, once again, your ability to fall asleep and stay asleep by re-
creating a positive connection between your bedroom and sleep.
As a first step, please ask yourself how you would feel about getting
up out of bed and leaving the bedroom whenever you have difficulty
falling asleep or staying asleep? Your answer to this question may
shed light on your personal view of your sleep problem, so it may be
worth pondering for a moment. We shall explore many such
questions throughout the book.

2

SLEEPY OR TIRED? — KNOW THE DIFFERENCE

QUICK GUIDE

Problem: Your ability to distinguish between genuine sleepiness and the feeling of fatigue or tiredness has become blurred, creating confusion about when to attempt to sleep.

Cause: You no longer experience the natural sequence of feeling first tired, then sleepy before dozing off.

Solution: Ask yourself during the day: "am I sleepy?" or "am I tired?" until you appreciate the distinction, then monitor these feelings near your bedtime.

Do you know the difference between feeling sleepy and feeling tired? This distinction may seem obvious to some yet unclear to others. The distinction, however, is a critical one for someone who suffers from insomnia.

Have you ever found yourself sitting quietly after lunch, and then noticed a strong feeling that you might doze off?

That's true sleepiness. When you feel sleepy, there is a definite sense of drowsiness that is quite pleasurable. Your body slumps into a state of relaxation and your mind drifts away from wakefulness into a hazier consciousness. If you stay awake or work while you are sleepy, a constant struggle ensues between the sleepiness that signals the pleasure to be gained from sleep and your attempt to remain alert. A battle line is drawn across which two opposing forces tug at you. And, at the end of the day, if sleepiness wins out, the genuine pleasure of falling asleep proves to be one of life's most consistently satisfying experiences.

Fatigue or tiredness is very different than sleepiness. Your body and mind feel worn out or overused. When you are fatigued but must continue to work, there is a constant sense of nagging in the back of your mind or discomfort permeating through the muscles of your body. There is no pleasure involved in feeling tired unless you can stop what you're doing and allow yourself some rest. Even then, rest may be unrewarding if you have the belief that what you really need is sleep, yet slumber will not come or is not permitted.

In the overwhelming majority of instances, it is essential to expect that sleepiness *precedes* and facilitates sleep; whereas, fatigue or tiredness may have a very inconsistent relationship to your ability to fall asleep.

As we move down the path toward healthy sleep, all the things we talk about and teach will be geared toward helping you to appreciate and regain your natural ability to feel sleepy. Once you trust this feeling of sleepiness, healthy sleep patterns can be reestablished more easily.

As another step in that direction, take a moment right now and ask yourself these questions:

Do I feel sleepy?

Do I feel tired?

Do I feel alert?

You probably recognize that there are instances in which you feel each of these three conditions separately, and in various combinations, and that is normal. But, it will prove valuable to permit yourself the opportunity to tease out these feelings and sensations in more specific ways. Near bedtime, for example, if you can appreciate that you feel more sleepy than alert, there's an excellent chance you can *let* yourself fall asleep. On the other hand, as bedtime approaches if you notice that you feel more tired than sleepy, it may prove more difficult to try to sleep; in fact, it may be counterproductive to even attempt sleep.

If you feel tired, particularly if your fatigue has been generated by an active lifestyle of work and/or play, then sleepiness should follow. That a sleepy feeling does not follow on the footsteps of fatigue is what goes to the heart of most insomnia problems. For some reason, this natural next step in the sequence — fatigue to sleepiness — does not occur. Your mind or your body (usually both) has learned to fight this progression; instead, you maintain a feeling of tiredness that no longer permits the pleasure of drowsiness to herald the need and desire for sleep.

When you learn to let tiredness take its natural course to

sleepiness, your effort is almost 99% complete — sleep is not far off.

Unless you have suffered from lifelong, night after night insomnia (which is rare by the way), at some point you must have engaged in normal and successful sleep habits. As such, there is likely to have been at least a few times in your life when you felt sleepiness as a natural thing prior to sleep. Nodding off was easy and a genuine pleasure. During these times, this natural ability promoted a very strong and healthy connection between sleep and your bedroom.

With insomnia, from whatever the cause, this once healthy association becomes weaker and inconsistent. Therefore, I would ask you again to imagine how it might feel to get up out of bed and leave the bedroom if you noticed you were feeling tired but not sleepy. This approach can be attempted regardless of whether the difficulty occurs at bedtime or in the middle of the night.

Conversely, if you *only* feel tired while attempting to doze off, you will most likely continue to weaken your connection to the bedroom as a place for slumber. When you consider this sleep hygiene approach, recognize that by leaving the bedroom on the occasion of sleeplessness, you may be able to take the cause of your insomnia *out* of the bedroom and leave it *outside* where it can no longer interfere with your sleep.

3

MAKE YOUR BEDROOM
SLEEPER-FRIENDLY

QUICK GUIDE

Problem: You can fall asleep in other rooms, even other homes or hotels, but not in your own bed or bedroom.

Cause: You have "learned" several negative associations between your *own* bed and other waking behaviors that condition you to remain awake in your *own* bedroom.

Solution: Use your bedroom only for sleep and nothing else until you consistently feel sleepy prior to bedtime.

◆ ◆ ◆

If you ate pizza late in the evening and then had a nightmare after going to bed, would you wonder if this snack had something to do with your disturbing dream? Some people speculate about these types of connections more than others, but what if the next week, you ate pizza again and had another bad dream. Your tendency to wonder if the two things were connected would likely increase.

Now suppose you ate pizza a third time over this short time span; it would be easy to imagine that you might have more than a passing thought about what you would dream that night. Suppose you had another nightmare — is the pizza to blame?

The answer is a definite yes and no.

There is no scientific evidence that pizza has any impact whatsoever on your dreams (thank goodness!). However, once your mind draws an association between pizza and bad dreams, just a single bite can stimulate thoughts and feelings in your waking consciousness that will trigger unpleasant dreams while asleep. The pizza serves as a stimulus or trigger, not because of anything in the ingredients, but simply because the image or the taste of pizza draws your memory back to the previous experiences with nightmares. In other words, a connection has been formed between pizza and nightmares.

The connections you develop between your ability to fall asleep and your sleep environment ultimately determine your success in achieving healthy sleep. At a younger age, most of your associations developed naturally. You didn't spend much time, if any, thinking about what to do to get to sleep:

In most instances, you felt tired, then sleepy, and then you went to sleep.

Over the course of your life, usually during times of stress, you learned new associations that conflict with these natural tendencies toward good sleep. These new associations represent negative connections, some more conscious than others, that weaken your confidence about your sleep habits.

The primary negative association, conscious or otherwise, is the belief that your bed and bedroom are no longer an obvious place to go to sleep and stay asleep. This association can be so strong that even if you start feeling very sleepy in the living room, you will come to full alertness when you walk into your bedroom. As a consequence, sooner or later, you may find yourself falling asleep in different places in your house, like the living room sofa or in the family room watching TV.

In time, you will feel tremendously frustrated if you feel sleepy in one part of your home, only to discover that this pleasurable feeling can be replaced in your bedroom in the blink of an eye with a sudden surge of alertness. More than frustrating, it is sometimes maddening, especially if you've spent a very active day at work or at play and feel you've earned a good night of slumber.

You most certainly do deserve a good night of sleep — many in fact — so hang in there and consider the following:

If you find yourself able to fall asleep in another room of the house, yet have difficulty doing so in your own bedroom, it is almost certain that you've developed a primary problem initiating sleep due to negative associations. When I interview patients with insomnia, one of the first questions I ask is if they've been on a vacation recently or spent the night at someone else's home. Often, someone who complains of not being able to fall asleep in his or her own bed will report no difficulty in dozing off in a hotel or at a friend's house.

Now, if we examine this person's insomnia in more depth with a polysomnogram — an all night laboratory test to evaluate one's sleep — this type of insomnia, that is, a delay in falling asleep, may never reveal itself because the new laboratory environment does not hold the same negative associations for the insomniac. It is quite common, and perhaps embarrassingly so, for the patient to awaken from the lab and admit that she never slept so well in recent memory.

So, if you can fall asleep in one place, but dread your own bed, how do you fix this?

Do you remember as a child or some other time when you played with a little straw toy called the Chinese Finger Puzzle. You inserted a finger from each hand into the ends of the short straw tube, but as you probably remember, the more you tugged at each end, the harder it became to remove your fingers. In fact, only when you relaxed your fingers and stopped trying so hard would they release from the tube. In effect, you learned how to *let* your fingers escape.

With insomnia, it is crucial to stop trying so hard to fall asleep. It will happen if you let it, but you can improve your chances by bringing genuine sleepiness back to the bedroom where it belongs. If you feel sleepy, remain there and let yourself doze off in your own bed. Consider leaving the bedroom temporarily, if in about thirty or forty minutes (just estimate, don't watch the clock) you've not fallen asleep. Whenever sleepiness returns, go back to bed. By doing so, you will re-build the positive connection between sleep and the bedroom that will help you rediscover your natural ability to fall asleep.

Finally, I'd like to mention something here about staying asleep. Some people can fall asleep without much difficulty, but then awaken in the middle of the night. They believe that their problem is in staying asleep, but I would suggest that the true problem remains that of falling asleep.

The reason that "returning to sleep" may be the more helpful view of the problem is that *everyone* awakens from sleep throughout the night and with some regularity. Good sleepers, however, have little difficulty dozing off again whether or not they recall their awakenings, which by the way, could easily number five or ten such episodes per hour or more.

While there may be numerous causes for awakenings that may need to be investigated, much of the time it is more practical and useful to still think of middle of the night insomnia as difficulty in falling asleep. Virtually all the tips that I will advise you on apply to both falling asleep at bedtime and in the middle of the night.

4

TIME IS NOT OF THE ESSENCE

QUICK GUIDE

Problem: Unwitting alerting behaviors are disrupting your ability to fall asleep or stay asleep.

Cause: Commonplace negative associations have developed such as looking at the clock to monitor how long it's taking you to fall asleep or how much sleep you anticipate getting.

Solution: Turn the clock to face the wall or remove the clock from the bedroom.

◆ ◆ ◆

Any negative associations between sleep and bedroom may seem challenging to deal with, yet in practicality, they are easy to solve because the solution is as simple as:

USING YOUR BEDROOM ONLY FOR SLEEP . . .

. . . OR MAKING LOVE.

Perhaps you think you are already doing this, but there are many subtle ways of defeating this singular principle. A prime example is clock-watching. If you are disturbed or frustrated by the length of time it takes to fall asleep, you may be the type of person who wishes to monitor exactly how much sleep you're losing. Or, if you awaken in the middle of the night, you may have developed the habit of turning over to see what time it is, so that you can calculate how much possible sleep time remains...if you could get back to sleep.

In both instances, your brain is engaged in an alerting type of behavior. When else do you look at the clock? Perhaps to check the time to: get to work? get to school? break for lunch? make an appointment? watch a favorite TV program? The list goes on. Checking the clock and thinking about time is a common waking behavior that occurs all day long and often right up until bedtime when you might check to see how late it is before retiring.

Looking at a clock, then, has a very strong association with activity and schedules and all sorts of hustle and bustle. It has everything to do with *not* falling asleep or staying asleep! Yet, given this knowledge, many insomniacs continue to monitor the clock and in so doing continue to fuel their insomnia.

So let's take a moment to look at the cognitions associated with time and clock-watching to figure out why it may be difficult for the insomnia sufferer to turn the clock to face the wall.

The prevailing view about time and sleep is that sleep quantity is the most important thing to measure. Why do we think this? One reason is that we have all been led down the garden path by being repeatedly told we're supposed to get 8 hours of sleep per night. Thus, anything fewer than 8 hours is going to make you feel like you must be coming up short. In actuality, the quantity of your sleep can't hold a candle to the importance of the *quality* of your sleep, and we'll talk more about that concept in ensuing chapters.

The bottom line then about time is that we have developed some beliefs about its relationship to sleep. If you are overly concerned about the amount of sleep you are supposed to get, then it makes perfect sense to want to count the minutes in the middle of the night and calculate the number of hours you might potentially obtain. So, not only does time mess up your sleep by having you spend time counting and not sleeping, but time pervades your whole perspective about sleep and sets you up for failure.

Time issues reflect even deeper concerns and fears about our lives. On a profound note, the questions that lurk within each of us, might be: Will I have enough time to accomplish all that I want to with my life? How much time do I really have to accomplish these things? On a pragmatic scale, there is the constant hurry-and-worry lifestyle that has infected modern society, such that instead of the old saw, "less is more", we now have a new mantram, "more is more." In truth, there is only so much that you can pack into any single day, and if you fail to meet your daily objectives, it is not uncommon to bring all that unsatisfied energy with you into the bedroom where you might mistakenly believe you can "finish your work."

Such an attitude completely negates the purpose of the bed and bedroom and of sleep itself. In this hectic and frazzled world, good sleep is not only necessary, but it is also a well-deserved break from our incredibly busy, hurry-and-worry lives. The bedroom therefore ought to become a type of sanctuary, a special place to shut out and turn off the misery and hassles of the world. Instead, it ought to be a place to tune in to the restorative and healing power of sleep.

Finally, clock watching is one of the best examples of how to engage in a behavior that foils your efforts to sleep because, in fact, you are *not* USING YOUR BEDROOM ONLY FOR SLEEP. While it might seem like a ludicrously simple treatment, I have helped some individuals completely overcome their sleeplessness by asking them to turn their clock to face the wall or to remove it altogether from the bedroom. No other therapy was required — the insomnia departed once they stopped checking the time.

If insomnia clock watching is a strong component of your nightly routine, it's likely you've been doing it for a long time. Regardless of how long you've engaged in time-checking, eliminating this alerting behavior from your bedroom can be a major step forward in your recovery of good sleep. Before proceeding, however, it is imperative to appreciate the connections you've developed between time and sleep. Once these associations are clearer to you, you will find it easier to turn the clock to the wall or to cover its face.

5

KILL YOUR TELEVISION

QUICK GUIDE

Problem: Television used to help you fall asleep, but now it no longer makes you feel drowsy.

Cause: Despite the boring programs on the tube, you have become accustomed to lying in bed to watch TV instead of lying in bed to sleep.

Solution: Do not watch TV in the bedroom.

◆ ◆ ◆

In treating insomnia with the principles of sleep hygiene, there are innumerable possibilities for negative connections that may need to be addressed; and, it is well worth your while to investigate all of them as each may serve as a cue that blocks your natural sleepiness. As we explore these major and minor situations, behaviors and so forth, please bear in mind that virtually all these considerations relate back to the singular problem of having learned to use your bedroom for something other than sleeping.

An area that would seem rather obvious as a potential problem has only recently (during the last forty years or so) entered into the realm of major obstacles to sound sleep — the television. TV has its own intrinsic drawbacks because it produces a passive relationship between the viewer and the tube, whereas other forms of activity yield a clearer sense of engaging in something of genuine benefit, be it work or play oriented.

While this passive effect of television can produce drowsiness in some people, by and large, TV is something you attempt to do as a waking behavior: you seek to watch your favorite program, or to see a sporting event with a group of friends or to catch up on the latest soap opera melodrama.

Therefore, if you watch TV in your bedroom, it is likely to disrupt your healthy sleep habits. At first, TV could help you feel drowsy, particularly because of the incredibly boring programs that now grace the airwaves; but, unfortunately, over time, TV will have the same impact as the clock. You are watching instead of sleeping, and your brain learns that the bed is no longer simply for slumber.

Once your mind establishes this connection, regardless of what you watch on TV, you have invoked an association that prevents your natural sleepiness. Again, it is this type of association, more than any other, that goes to the heart of the problem, that is, your unconscious continues to receive a mixed message: watch TV and sleep, just like watch the clock and sleep. The conflict hidden in these mixed signals festers in your mind without much awareness, yet it wreaks havoc on your sleep.

Television can also play an active role in disrupting your sleep if you happen to watch over-stimulating newscasts or sex and action programming. These shows bring anyone to full attention, and some of the more horrific stories disrupt your sleep in more direct fashion by producing disturbing dreams. Self-serving, selfish and brazenly dishonest TV producers continue to attempt to discredit the research that demonstrates quite clearly that TV pictures will implant images into your mind, but both common sense and the facts speak otherwise.

In my own research specialty of helping people with chronic nightmares, I have learned that those afflicted with frequent bad dreams will limit the amount of television they watch. They do so for the obvious reason to prevent the influx of disturbing images that will then trigger a new round of nightmares.

Last, TV also plays havoc with your circadian rhythm — the body's natural biological clock — that gears you up in the morning for a full day of activity and winds you down in the evening to prepare you for sleep. Television interferes with this biological rhythm by encouraging you to stay up later. While most adults will have the first sensation of sleepiness somewhere close to 9:00 PM or earlier, TV induces people to remain awake for hours beyond that time frame. For normal sleepers, this is likely to produce a routine cycle of insufficient sleep, but for insomniacs it can throw a monkey wrench into their circadian rhythm by teaching them to remain awake past midnight and thereby exacerbate their existing difficulty with falling asleep. Eventually, the combination of late-night TV and insomnia can produce an entirely new circadian rhythm of going to sleep in the wee hours of the night, which can reduce the insomniac's already shortened sleep cycle to dramatically low levels.

Television's effects on sleep are marked and omnipresent in our society. Learning how to limit the use of TV and removing the TV from the bedroom are two of the healthiest steps you can take in promoting good sleep hygiene and sound sleep. As a fallback maneuver, if you have a VCR, you can always consider videotaping a favorite late night show and watching it outside the bedroom at a more convenient time.

6

YOU'VE MADE YOUR BED, BUT DON'T SUFFER IN IT

QUICK GUIDE

Problem: You spend a long time in bed lying awake either when you try to fall asleep or in the middle of the night.

Cause: You have developed the ultimate negative connection between your bed and mental alertness — you have programmed yourself to stay awake and not sleep in the bedroom.

Solution: Never spend more than a set, estimated period in bed awake (for example, twenty or forty or sixty minutes); if you're not asleep when the estimated time is up, leave the bedroom and return when you feel sleepy.

◆ ◆ ◆

Reading in bed fits into a special category because it can help or hinder your ability to fall asleep. Some people swear by their use of light reading material in bed just a few minutes before lights out. Others feel enough stimulation to find themselves reading two hours later!

Your decision about whether to read in bed or not must be weighed with your practical experience. If it works, even though it would appear to fly in the face of the general principles of sleep hygiene, perhaps it is helping you to relax and take your mind off the day's events or future worries. If it doesn't work and merely exacerbates your difficulties with falling asleep, then it is probably stimulating and alerting you and thwarting your natural sleepiness. *Outside of the bedroom*, however, reading is probably one of the single best activities you can do as you await the return of drowsiness.

While television, clock watching, and reading at length represent the most common negative associations that could interfere with falling asleep and staying asleep, there are many others that also may need to be addressed. If you use your bedroom as an office for paying bills, can you imagine what a bad connection this would build as you literally let financial stress and worries into your bed? Writing letters in bed may be another negative influence unless you use a diary or a journal to unwind from the day's events. So, all these kinds of behaviors must be examined, including speaking on the telephone or whatever else you find yourself doing on the bed instead of sleeping or making love.

Of all the possible negative situations, though, the simplest *and* worst for your sleep is **lying awake in bed**.

A TV, phone, clock or a book are external, physical objects that occupy your attention, prohibiting your natural tendency toward sleep; but, it is ultimately the internal processes of your mind and body that determine whether or not you can shut off the day's events so that drowsiness eventually leads to sleep. If you choose to remain in bed *and* think, you are establishing the strongest possible connection between your bed and mental activity and alertness. In other words, your bedroom becomes a place no longer associated with sleeping; instead, your bed itself becomes a place to continue the day's events in your mind's eye.

Just as you would not, at least knowingly, go to your workplace to sleep, why would you enter your sleep-place to work?

This negative mental connection between bedroom and thinking is perhaps the most difficult habit to overcome for any insomniac, particularly because someone who suffers from sleeplessness may stay in bed for any number of reasons, all of which appear to be quite reasonable.

Most people assume that it's better to rest even if you can't get to sleep. Others can't imagine getting up out of bed because all they really want to do is sleep. Those who lie in bed with racing thoughts often feel powerless to stop them. Then, there are those who lie awake apparently without any thoughts whatsoever, but still they feel frozen to the mattress.

Yet, in response to this wide assortment of reasons for remaining awake in bed, sleep hygiene offers one simple challenge: GET UP OUT OF BED AND LEAVE THE BEDROOM UNTIL YOU FEEL SLEEPY!

This is the cornerstone of sleep hygiene. And, while this specific advice seems to be a difficult pill to swallow, especially during the first few trials, it has proven time and again to be the single most effective component of any sleep promoting regimen for someone suffering from insomnia.

The advice to get up out of bed and leave the bedroom may sound drastic, but the connection that your mind has made between sleep and wakefulness is exceedingly powerful. In no uncertain terms, to lie awake in bed, whether you think, don't think, rest or don't rest, your mind and body now believe that the bed and the bedroom are places in which it's perfectly normal to remain awake . . . and suffer the distress of insomnia!

When you leave the bedroom and engage in some activity in another room — reading, writing, eating a small snack, or even watching TV — you have begun the reprogramming process of letting your mind know that wakefulness occurs outside the bedroom, *not* in the bed. This new and healthier habit can be learned in a matter of days, sometimes a mere three days.

To repeat, the key is to let your natural sleepiness reassert itself so that you return to the bedroom only when you feel drowsy. Then, if you were to lie down, but the sensation of wakefulness returned, you would be faced with the same challenge as before, that is, you would need to leave the bedroom yet again. To some, this may prove very frustrating, especially because this process may need repeating several times in the first few nights. These initial attempts, as challenging as they may appear, will often produce rapid success in learning to overcome the unhealthy habit of lying awake in bed.

In practice, suppose you had to get up out of bed and leave the bedroom not just once or twice, but three times? Can you imagine how taxing it would be to your sense of well-being? It might seem like you were adding to your efforts to get to sleep. Fortunately, there is nothing harmful about this routine. More to the point, it is essential that you realize that lying in bed awake is what is really harmful if your goal is to fall asleep; moreover, lying in bed awake for a lengthy time is rarely restful.

For example, if you had the choice of lying in bed for only six and one-half hours with a guarantee that you would always sleep six hours, or you could lie in bed for ten hours with no guarantee of how many hours you might sleep, which routine would you choose?

Your answer will tell you a lot about your own understanding of sleep and rest.

7

QUALITY, NOT QUANTITY

QUICK GUIDE

Problem: Your sleep is light, superficial and unrestful.

Cause: Your total time in bed involves too much time awake, which then filters into your unconscious to fragment your actual sleep.

Solution: Focus on sleep quality, not quantity. Less time in bed will retrain your mind to facilitate deeper sleep.

◆ ◆ ◆

If it surprises you that the person who spends *less* time in bed will have better quality sleep, then please consider this related example: two people both receive exactly six hours of sleep each night, but one lies in bed ten hours while the other spends only six and one-half hours there.

Will the six hours of sleep be the same for each person?

Most likely not. Perhaps you wonder why six hours sleep

isn't the same six hours in either case. Please let me expand on this so it will help you further realize the importance of not remaining in bed while awake.

Sleep, as we understand it with the relatively primitive technological tools we have at our disposal, appears to progress through a variety of stages during the course of a normal night's sleep. In non-medical terms, it is easiest to describe these as three types: deep sleep, light sleep and dream awareness sleep.

When a person is studied in a sleep lab with the polysomnogram, she is hooked up to numerous wires, probes and monitors to measure brain waves, eye movements, breathing, snoring, chin tension, heart rate, chest, abdominal and leg movements. By monitoring all this information, we can establish how much time you spend in the various sleep stages.

For most insomniacs, an inordinate amount of time is usually spent in the lighter stages of sleep at the expense of both deep and dream awareness sleep. As you might imagine, the lack of adequate deep and dream stages partially explains why an insomniac often complains of feeling unrested. This complaint is legitimate and can easily be reproduced by anyone who attempts to sleep an entire night with loud and irritating music or other noises close to the bedside.

In other words, if you sleep *lightly* much of the time — which unfortunately is standard for the insomniac — then the actual number of total hours slept may be meaningless to you.

From numerous medical-scientific research investigations, it can be clearly stated that:

The longer you remain in bed in a vain attempt to sleep, the more you will disrupt your overall sleep by limiting the amount of deep and dream sleep.

The reason for this paradox is that the longer you remain in bed, you are likely to be experiencing an increase in the amount of time awake. In the field of sleep medicine, we call this *sleep fragmentation* because you alternate between sleep and brain arousals or full awakenings.

For example, even if you slept six hours while lying in bed for ten, you will have also experienced four hours of wakefulness. For reasons that are not completely understood, it appears that this increase in time awake (the four hours) filters into your unconscious during your time asleep (the six hours). By repeating this process nightly, your mind distinguishes less and less between **being asleep and being awake.** The result is that your sleep cycle spends more time in the lighter stages. At some point, your sleep can become so superficial, you may think you're not even sleeping at all or perhaps for just a few hours.

Sadly, this very well-intentioned attempt to gain sufficient hours of slumber almost always yields lighter sleep, and as you futilely attempt to spend more time in bed, the vicious cycle continues or worsens.

The old saying — "less is more" — speaks volumes to anyone suffering from insomnia, particularly those who have been troubled chronically by sleeplessness.

Sleep quality is the crucial factor in helping the insomniac to rehabilitate herself. Once you learn to focus on the quality of sleep, even slight increases in your deep or dream sleep will usher in an entirely new and decidedly more satisfying perspective regarding your ability to obtain restful and refreshing slumber.

If you currently spend more than one or two hours in bed awake, then consider cutting this down 15 minutes per night for a week. Then, the second week cut it another 15 minutes per night, and so on, each week until you are spending less than one total hour awake in bed. Some people can cut down their time in bed more rapidly, which is fine if you are eager to attempt such a drastic approach. It has been known to work "miracles." For others who want to change at a slower pace, I recommend the more gradual approach, but please note that your results will come more gradually as well. In sum, decreased time in bed will generate sounder sleep, particularly if you can decrease your time awake in bed to less than one hour.

Remember, in this instance *less* really is *more*.

8

OVERCOMING THE FEAR OF INSOMNIA

QUICK GUIDE

Problem: You cannot get to sleep because you worry about not getting to sleep — you are afraid you might be harming your health if you don't gain sufficient rest.

Cause: Fear has many disguises: insomnia and fears about sleeplessness are a very common one.

Solution: Recognize that no one has ever died from a loss of sleep; but also take time to examine other fears in your life — work stress, relationship conflicts, other health concerns. These may be the real sources of the fear that you have developed about insomnia.

◆ ◆ ◆

Does a shorter time in bed mean that the insomniac is doomed to a life of shorter sleep? By all means no!

But the practice of a shorter sleep cycle may be worthwhile

during specific episodes of insomnia, and it may teach you how <u>not</u> to worry about your total sleep. Moreover, by appreciating the importance of sleep quality, you may shift your focus away from your worries about overall sleep time.

The worries that people develop about their sleep habits are genuine and often very emotional. The two most common feelings are the fear that you will not be able to fall asleep and the fear that you will be harmed by not obtaining enough sleep.

Let's examine both these fears.

It is helpful to understand that no one has ever died directly from a lack of sleep. There is an extremely rare hereditary disorder known as Fatal Familial Insomnia, but this disease is related to severe brain degeneration, which causes the sleeplessness, not the reverse.

To be sure, people who suffer chronic insomnia may be vulnerable to infectious illness like colds or the flu, or they may be prone to accidents, errors and mistakes, such as motor vehicle accidents or lapses in concentration or memory while home or at work; however, any specific night of lost or reduced sleep is not likely to be directly harmful in a manner that could cause life-threatening health problems like heart attacks or strokes.

Despite hearing the above explanation, I know from my clinical practice that some people with insomnia retain a fear of sleeplessness that may become irrational. I therefore want to reiterate two points if you still fear that insomnia may cause you serious physical harm.

First, insomnia itself cannot directly cause you any injury. People in all walks of life experience occasional episodes of sleeplessness because of situations related to work, school, children crying in the night, or other events. Some of these people are faced with regularly occurring episodes of sleep deprivation similar to some insomniacs. Commonly, these people respond to lost sleep by attempting to go about the next day's business, perhaps with greater fatigue, or by using caffeinated beverages, or by trying to catch a nap later in the day. Further, there have been no scientific reports showing that a single lost night of sleep results in serious harm. Of course, after a lost night of sleep, it certainly would be more prudent to avoid driving a car on a long-distance solo excursion, or to avoid other potentially dangerous situations.

Second, when a person develops an irrational fear about sleep, there is invariably some other fear that is lurking beneath the surface that has been displaced into a fear about insomnia. In my experience, deep-seated emotions — typically disturbing ones, such as depression, anxiety, guilt, or anger — are often the underlying culprits that are the real cause of fear.

Depression can be a brutal and agonizing experience, inflicting more pain and misery than almost the worst imaginable physical pain. With physical pain there may appear to be some chance that at some point the problem will resolve. With serious depression, often the individual feels hopeless—the future appears bleak without any promise of recovery. For these reasons, a person might grow to fear depression, especially if she has experienced it once and dreads the day she might be depressed again. In some instances, then, a person who has developed an irrational fear of insomnia because of deeper emotional distress may need counseling of some sort to help connect and deal with the real fear.

The fear of not being able to fall asleep may fit into the

same category. Insomniacs who reach a state of exasperation will often describe an intense frustration that arises in the bedroom when they attempt to doze. Again, this fear may be the sign of emotional turmoil. A classic case would be the individual who has been noticing stress at work. Anticipation of renewed conflict on a particular day may spark a genuine fear about returning to work; this fear is then displaced into a fear about not being able to go to sleep.

Some of these emotionally charged situations can be discussed with an attentive and compassionate person, such as a health care professional or a minister. Often, your primary doctor or a sympathetic clergyman would be the place to start although short term counseling from a mental health therapist could also produce dramatic improvement in your ability to cope with the underlying conflict.

With respect to sleep hygiene, it's important to realize that irrational fears about insomnia are likely to thwart your straightforward efforts to reprogram your sleep patterns. On the other hand, it's also of benefit to recognize that the simple solutions offered through a sleep hygiene program may breathe enough confidence into your attitude to assist you in overcoming these troublesome fears.

It must also be stated, however, that if you have a real fear for your safety in your sleep environment, then it is incumbent upon you to find a way to improve the situation as best you can. No one should ever tell you to downplay such a fear, for when you are asleep, you may be extremely vulnerable if someone or something were to pose a threat to you. In this instance, it is essential that you take measures to enhance your safety. This might include getting better locks on doors and windows, installing a security alarm, having a guard dog, or having good friends and neighbors who know your concerns and will check up on you. In some situations, while it may sound extreme to some (you must be the judge), a weapon of some sort may be what ultimately makes you feel secure in your bedroom.

Last, if you have experienced too many bad nights to count, you may develop a fear about any single bad night's sleep. That is, you now believe that regaining your healthy sleep is an all-or-nothing affair; unless you sleep well every night, one bad night will trigger weeks or months of insomnia. Not only is this view unrealistic, but it is also counterproductive. Everyone—good sleepers included—has some bad nights. Unfortunately, your memory of too many bad nights may cloud this perception of normal sleep. So, as your insomnia improves, please keep in mind that a bad night of sleep does not have to produce a domino effect.

9

DOES YOUR SCHEDULE NEED A WAKE-UP CALL?

QUICK GUIDE

Problem: Your difficulty in falling asleep creates havoc with your life's schedule because you can fall asleep far beyond your normal bedtime, and then find yourself sleeping later the next day.

Cause: Your natural biological clock—the circadian rhythm—is being pushed beyond its normal schedule.

Solution: Pick a set wakeup time and follow it seven days per week (allow no more than a one hour difference on the weekends) even if you stay up late some nights.

Now let's return to bedtime and wakeup schedules — the Benjamin Franklin approach to sound slumber and another key to sleep hygiene. We've mentioned circadian rhythms — the body's biological timekeeper. Once you understand the general nature of your circadian rhythm, you can use this information to build a schedule that promotes better sleep. In acknowledging the value of your innate biological clock, you will note once again the emphasis on sleep quality over total sleep time.

The circadian rhythm naturally establishes a pattern of being awake during the day and being asleep during the night.

A substantial inducement to this pattern is that your body's temperature rises and remains higher during the day; whereas, at night, your body temperature falls and remains low. Both the difference in temperature, that is, between higher and lower, and the changing nature of the temperature, that is, rising and falling, are linked to your ability to be awake and stay awake and to your ability to fall asleep and stay asleep, respectively.

Anything that promotes a consistent day-night rhythm yields a similar consistency in these temperature patterns that will facilitate alertness and sleepiness at appropriate times. The easiest way to help your body maintain a consistent rhythm is by establishing regular bedtimes and wakeup times.

For most insomniacs, a regular bed and wakeup schedule would be very satisfying. Unfortunately, once the sleeplessness kicks in, your efforts to maintain a schedule are often thwarted. It is not uncommon for insomniacs to wait later and later in the night to get to bed because they fear that they will fail in their attempt to fall asleep. If sleep does not commence until the early morning, they may doze well beyond their normal wakeup time. This delay in falling asleep and waking up indicates to your body that the time for going to bed is progressively later and the hour for waking up is later, too.

This cycle of delay can become so chronic that some poor sleepers think that they are now "night people" who can only go to sleep in the middle of the night or the early morning hours. In fact, they are partially right because their bodies' circadian rhythms may be entrained or patterned after this night owl schedule.

Changing such a rhythm takes time and can be frustrating, but what's even more difficult to change is a rhythm that jumps all around the clock when an insomniac's lifestyle becomes helter-skelter. In either of these two situations where the body's rhythm has deviated far from the norm, it is usually more helpful for the patient to seek help from a sleep disorders specialist. A physician or psychologist who specializes in sleep medicine will have training and clinical experience in managing the individual's recovery to a normal rhythm.

Most insomniacs do not reach this severe level of circadian disturbance; however, periodically they will notice enough variation in their sleep cycle to cause sporadic bed and wakeup times, which may be further compounded by erratic napping. Other examples of this problem would be staying up late or sleeping late on weekends, which will then influence the weekday schedule along a similar track.

Since most insomniacs complain about falling asleep as their primary problem, trying to establish a regular bedtime is likely to be a nonstarter. Instead, the sensible strategy is to work "backwards" by committing to a regular wakeup time. If you can establish this morning time *seven days per week*, it will produce enough regularity to eventually influence your bedtime.

Let's use the example of a 7:00 AM wakeup time. About an hour or more before 7:00 AM, your body has actually begun reheating itself, that is, your body temperature is beginning to rise after having fallen most of the night. Therefore, if you awaken at seven o'clock with or without an alarm, you are engaging in a pattern very consistent with the body's desire to wake up.

Combining this wake up time with the fundamental sleep hygiene principle to use the bedroom only for sleep means that once seven o'clock arrives, you want to get up out of bed as soon as is reasonably possible (preferably within ten minutes) and leave the bedroom once you've finished with the bathroom, dressing and so forth.

When you attempt this scheduling technique, do not be discouraged if this regular wakeup time does not produce an immediate impact on your bedtime. Given a fair trial and notwithstanding the old adage, don't be surprised if you discover that the tail can indeed wag the dog.

10

ADDING MORE QUALITY
TO YOUR SLEEP

QUICK GUIDE

Problem: You want to sleep eight hours per night, but you only appear to be getting six.

Cause: Your focus on sleep quantity has led you to believe that the actual number of hours you sleep will determine how well you will feel in the morning.

Solution: Re-evaluate your expectations so that you can improve sleep quality first and let quantity take care of itself.

For starters, a regular morning wakeup time coupled to a quick exit from the bedroom sends a very powerful sleep hygiene message to the brain. In effect, you are letting your mind know two things. One is that wakefulness is separated from sleep because you've adopted the "up and at 'em" mindset. The other is that you have linked your wakefulness to the body's natural biological timekeeper, which has been working to get you up anyway.

In time — often in just a matter of days or even less — this regular wakeup schedule can influence your bedtime, again for the same two reasons: that is, your body's circadian rhythm will start winding down toward nighttime; and, you've been out of bed all day keeping wakefulness separate from sleepiness.

If you do not get sleepy near to what you deem to be your proper bedtime, then we need to explore what this might mean. Say, for example, that you wake up at seven o'clock and therefore expect to go to bed by eleven at night so you can get the standard eight hours of sleep.

Is this realistic?

Maybe, maybe not.

The more appropriate question to ask first is what is the average number of hours of sleep you think you're getting currently?

If you know you're only getting six or seven hours, then you might pose the question: how realistic is it to think that you might suddenly jump back up to eight?

This leads us back to the same quantity vs. quality issues that compel us to declare:

If your average sleep is now six hours, then learning to capitalize on SIX GOOD HOURS OF SLEEP is the goal at hand.

Slowly, over time, perhaps these six hours can be extended *and* quality can be maintained. But attempting to do the reverse, that is, adding quantity initially is more likely to diminish quality. This is why we focus on quality, which on virtually every count is more important than sleep quantity.

Add quality to your sleep first!

So, if your regular bedtime remains inconsistent, the next thing we need to examine is your expectation about the total amount of sleep you believe you need. By honestly arriving at a clear picture of your average sleep time, you can use a similar number to enhance your sleep quality by selecting a conforming bedtime.

If you're now averaging six hours of sleep, you can add about thirty to sixty minutes to this total to come up with six and a half or seven hours of total time in bed. If you select seven hours of total bedtime and you have a wakeup time of 7:00 AM, then bedtime should be at midnight.

This might seem late if you've being trying to get into bed at ten o'clock. But, with an average of only six hours of slumber, you are probably fragmenting your sleep by confusing your mind and body with a prolonged amount of time in bed.

To summarize, you must determine the average amount of sleep you're now getting and then add about thirty to sixty minutes to that total to arrive at how much time to spend in bed. This will also assist you in determining a proper bed and wakeup time. If you extend your time in bed beyond this framework, your sleep is likely to become very inefficient, which brings us to the concept of sleep efficiency.

11

SLEEP PRESSURE INCREASES SLEEP EFFICIENCY

QUICK GUIDE

Problem: Your sleep efficiency is poor. Compared with the amount of time you spend in bed, you get too little sleep.

Cause: Your biological "sleep pressure" has been reduced by a number of habits that have blurred the natural distinction between your sleep and waking behaviors.

Solution: Consider reducing your total sleep time so that you never spend more than one-half hour awake in bed.

Did you know that the longer you remain awake, the greater your physiological drive for sleep? This is known as *sleep pressure*. In other words, the less you sleep, the greater your body's need for sleep. Certainly this makes sense, but did you also know that by increasing your sleep pressure, you can deepen your sleep as well? How then can an insomniac take advantage of this natural physiological response? The answer is to learn how to use sleep pressure to increase your *sleep efficiency.*

Sleep efficiency is your total sleep time (e.g. 9 hours) divided by your time in bed (e.g. 10 hours). These numbers are not equal because you must spend some time awake in bed if only a few minutes when you first lie down or upon awakening before getting up. Time in bed therefore is always longer than time asleep. In the above example, your sleep efficiency would equal 90% (9/10).

Most normal adult sleepers will demonstrate at least an 85% efficiency (6.75 hours sleep/8 hours in bed) in the sleep lab, and usually higher levels such as 90% (7.25 hours sleep/8 hours in bed) at home. Children often sleep with the highest efficiencies, sometimes reaching almost 95% efficiency (9.50 hours sleep/10 hours in bed).

Most insomniacs do not achieve these sleep efficiency percentages because of two fundamental problems. First, if you develop unrealistic expectations about falling asleep without being sleepy, then your total time in bed will increase as you lie awake in bed. Second, because so many insomniacs also suffer from light or interrupted sleep, there is a tendency to wake up at least once (if not many times) during the night and again lie awake in bed.

In talking about sleep pressure and efficiency we return to the concept of sleep quality. So, if you increase your sleep pressure, not only will your efficiency increase, but your overall quality will go up as well because you will restore some of your natural deep sleep. This improvement in quality can be realized in a matter of days (if not one night) by either shortening your time in bed, or by marginally restricting your amount of actual sleep.

I must say that I recognize that the concept of sleep pressure seems paradoxical to an insomniac because there is already a concern about getting too little sleep. This is a fair question because most poor sleepers do indeed receive insufficient sleep; why, then, would you want to consider getting even less?

While it might seem like harsh punishment to the insomniac, please bear in mind that a poor sleeper already has suffered an actual decrease in the total number of hours slept due to the fragmented slumber caused by excess time awake in bed. This light or disrupted sleep in insomnia is nearly universal; therefore, if increasing your sleep pressure yields deeper and more qualitatively restful sleep, then the final number of hours slept will be irrelevant compared with the immediate and real gains from improved sleep quality.

Sometimes, you will only need minor changes in your schedule to increase this natural sleep pressure and thus promote deeper, higher quality slumber. Moreover, the increase in pressure invariably renews the feeling of sleepiness at the end of the day that is sure to add to your confidence. When your natural desire to let yourself fall asleep regains a foothold at the appropriate time of your day-night cycle, you will reach a point where you no longer need to plan or worry about your sleeping habits. Instead, the whole process of sleeping will run its natural course as it once did earlier in your life when sleep was not a problem.

By temporarily producing a slight increase in your sleep pressure, you will foster better quality; and, over time, you may be able to expand your routine to a longer time in bed without sacrificing this quality. This is likely to occur if you have incorporated the basic sleep hygiene principle of separating sleep from wakefulness. Once your mind and body integrate this distinction into your schedule, then your sleep has a much greater opportunity to return to a more natural cycle; and, this cycle may prove to be a longer one coupled with higher quality.

12

A GREAT MATTRESS WILL
NOT LAST FOREVER

QUICK GUIDE

Problem: You do not sleep well on your current mattress.

Cause: Your mattress may be old and uncomfortable, but the larger problem, then, is that you now have a conditioned mistrust for your bedding which guarantees a poor night's sleep.

Solution: Buy a new mattress or improve your current one with supplemental foam pads and mattress covers.

◆ ◆ ◆

We have been focusing on the core sleep hygiene principles that must be addressed by essentially all who suffer from insomnia. At the heart of these principles is the singular distinction of learning to separate your sleep from your waking behaviors.

We have also discussed how seemingly minor conditions may provoke poor sleep by serving as major obstacles to your natural tendencies for sound slumber. Clock-watching is one example of a seemingly innocuous activity; yet, I hope that you can appreciate how dramatic an effect this behavior can have on your sleep, and how some people have literally cured their insomnia by removing the clock or turning it to face the wall.

I refer to this classic example again because it illustrates how a tiny obstacle on the road to sound sleep can veer you off course so easily. And yet many times, unwittingly, such a tiny obstacle will have been present for months or years before it will become clear to you that it is disturbing your sleep. The process is much like a splinter under your skin that causes constant irritation long before you might remove it. With this in mind, I want to spend time now reviewing a number of these so-called minor conditions so you can rectify those that may be interfering with your sleep.

An unsurprising example of a minor obstacle regards your mattress. Many people use a mattress for years partially because they are advertised to last for ten or twenty, but also because it is more expedient to keep using it. Good mattresses are not cheap and spending money to replace an old one does not appear convincingly cost-effective . . . at the moment.

How important is having the right mattress?

Let's ask it another way. Would you be comfortable sleeping on a hardwood floor? a lumpy sofa? or a short pile rug?

Probably not. Yet, when was the last time you investigated the condition, texture and comfort of your current mattress?

Your sleep is intimately connected to your mattress for the obvious reason that you must sleep on it. But, more importantly, if you have developed any mistrust about the quality and comfort of your bedding, can you imagine how readily this will filter into your unconscious? Conversely, imagine the positive influence it would have on your sleep to relish the thought of lying down on a mattress you know to be exceptionally comfortable.

Once again, we return to this process of connections. In this instance, it's not just that a mattress may be uncomfortable, it is more that your awareness of this discomfort will set you up — night after night — to expect poor quality or otherwise inadequate sleep. This relationship is so strong that if you were to use a substandard mattress, but believed you could sleep well on it, then you very well may do just that.

How do you determine if you have the right mattress? This is easy if you are open to the possibility that your mattress is not helping your sleep. All you must do is spend a few hours shopping at mattress stores. First, though, spend a good ten minutes or so lying on your own bed to test the comfort of your mattress. During this time, it will be helpful to let your thoughts drift a bit so that any feelings of discomfort about your bedding can come into your awareness. These are the kinds of thoughts and feelings that will inform you of how much you believe your mattress can or cannot affect your sleep.

If you have a good mattress and you're convinced it's not the problem, there is no need to purchase another one. If you are suspicious, but not sure, you certainly need to confer with your spouse or partner if you sleep together. If you sleep alone, then go shopping and make comparisons between your mattress and those at various stores.

How much to pay for bedding probably depends on how

high-tech you want to go. Sleep medicine is becoming an enormous field; as such, more companies are investigating new and beneficial ways of improving the utility of mattresses and other bedding components. Water beds, air cushioning, special new foam materials as well as advances in traditional coil structures will add great variety to your options. As always, you get what you pay for, yet don't hesitate to shop around as there are usually some savings to be gained if you don't rush out and buy the first brand. Finally, nowadays there are some long-term warranties that come with most mattresses to back up their longevity claims. A reliable guarantee — in writing — will help you get your money's worth.

13

THE ADVANTAGE OF A QUIET AND DARK BEDROOM

QUICK GUIDE

Problem: Excess light and noise disturb your sleep.

Cause: Environmental circumstances, for example, insensitive neighbors or other uncontrollable events, interfere with your sleep and worsen your insomnia.

Solution: Earplugs and nightshades should be a last resort. Talk with your neighbors while expecting to have to talk to them again . . . and again; do so candidly but without hostility: remember, if they don't have sleep problems, they do not understand your predicament. Be imaginative and consider a white noise device.

Would you knowingly try to fall asleep each night in a hot, brightly lit room with stale air, lots of dust, and loud, raucous music playing at your bedside?

Obviously not. To be sure, there are those who do not suffer from insomnia who can sleep like a log under such adverse conditions; but, for an insomniac, this scenario would be like putting out a fire with gasoline.

Your environment is another one of these seemingly minor conditions that can have profound consequences on your sleep if not attended to in a healthy manner.

Light, air, temperature, noise and cleanliness are crucial environmental factors and each person must determine what works best for them. More critically, however, because many normal sleepers tend to be insensitive to those with poor sleep, these issues require that the insomniac develop some assertiveness if it is other people or circumstances that disturb the sleep environment.

A completely dark room is the best possible sleep environment based solely on the physiologic responses of the human body. This does not account, though, for a person's need to feel safe and secure in the bedroom. Therefore, if a small amount of light — such as a plug-in night bulb — is required, that's fine. Keep in mind, though, if you are willing to experiment with a darker room, you may reap the benefits of placing your body in synch with the natural day-night cycle that promotes sleep. And, it's not that expensive to put up opaque window shades. Last, if you want the lights out, but circumstances are beyond your control, night shades can be worn over the eyes without much strain.

Noise reduction, unfortunately, is a much more complicated affair. First off, your last resort is earplugs, which only work up to a point unless you're willing to spend the money for custom fitted devices. Preferably, you'll never reach the point where you have to consider earplugs.

The problem of noise, however, is pervasive unless you live in a very rural environment, but then the chickens, pheasants, and other birds will get you early in the morning anyway. This pervasiveness is so dramatic in our so-called modern society that most people rarely experience what a long time ago used to be called "quiet" — the word and what it comprises do not really exist anymore in our communities. Even if you live in an exceptionally well insulated home to shield you from outside noises, inside rumblings from heating and cooling equipment and other appliances are very likely to disturb your sleep if you are very sensitive to noise as are many insomniacs.

Because good sleepers tend to be able to sleep anywhere, they have learned to adapt to the din of traffic noises, or the roar of planes overhead, or sirens, or loud parties, or barking dogs or whatever. To these relatively self-centered individuals, it is inconceivable that noise could somehow hamper someone else's sleep. These people can be so dense that if you told them they were making too much noise in their neighboring apartment, their immediate reaction would be gross confusion, followed usually by some low-level hostility.

This attitude is problematic because in dealing with noise issues you're weighing in directly against the grain of society. In our overstimulated environment, the majority of people allow their senses to deaden so that they can adapt to both chronic low grade noise as well as loud and raucous disturbances. There ought to be a law! In fact, there are many such laws that are on your side, but it is a delicate, if not touchy, encounter to assert your rights for a modicum of quiet.

I could recount numerous stories of both friends and patients where the cure proved worse than the disease, so hostile and upsetting was the response from their noisy neighbors. These insensitive responses led to more frustration and subsequently worse sleep from the build up of unvented irritation. And, all that they had asked was that someone simply turn down the volume.

Consider the possibility of honest discussion by offering to explain your difficulty with insomnia, but be prepared to lie, yes lie, or say anything to convince them of your need to sleep on a regular schedule. Tell them you get ear infections when you wear earplugs; tell them you're in school and you have to take a special exam every morning in class; tell them you're working eighty hours per week and you only get a chance to sleep five or six hours a night; tell them anything! They may or may not listen. You might also consider a mediation service, but then you would have to convince your neighbor to enter into such an arrangement.

When all else fails, seriously consider the concept of white noise. Although some insomniacs find this just as irritating, others find genuine relief with a well-placed fan or some other soothing sound-making device. This is usually less irritating than earplugs and certainly better than having to deal with the anticipation of your neighbor's or the surrounding communities incessant attacks on your eardrums.

14

FIND THE PROPER BEDROOM
TEMPERATURE

QUICK GUIDE

Problem: You want to sleep in fresh, clean air from an open window, but you feel more comfortable in a warm bedroom.

Cause: Insomniacs tend to feel chilly at bedtime because their skin temperature may be lower than normal.

Solution: Experiment with the proper mix of blankets, a fan and a cracked window. Consider a hot bath before bedtime. Aim for the fresh air approach, but defer to your need for a warm environment.

◆ ◆ ◆

From light and noise, we move on to fresh air, temperature and cleanliness.

A clean sleeping environment has two major benefits for you, one physical, the other mental. From a health standpoint, a clean bedroom will promote healthier breathing while you sleep.

The build up of dust, mites, molds and other allergens and irritants in the room, or worse in your bedding, will cause sneezing, coughing, and nasal congestion.

To sleep well, you need to breathe well.

This may require regular dusting and vacuuming as well as frequent linen changes. More so, a mattress cover can definitely serve as a barrier to particulate matter that might be harbored inside the mattress itself. Whether or not you need to explore hypoallergenic pillows or other such sheets and blankets is a matter of cost and personal preference.

Regardless of how you approach this matter, it is essential to feel a sense of comfort about sleeping in a clean bedroom. A dusty room that irritates your nose will deliver a strong message to the brain heralding the onset of less than optimal breathing while you sleep. Thus, the mental aspect of sleeping in an unclean room will eventually produce an association significant enough to prevent or disrupt your slumber.

Another consideration along these lines is the need for fresh air. Many people sleep with an open or cracked window all year long regardless of the weather. Notwithstanding the possibility of a greater exposure to allergens such as pollens, fresh air can promote a sense of cleanliness and thereby facilitate easier breathing.

While sleeping, it is useful to recognize that your body enters into a catabolic state, that is, because you are no longer eating or drinking, your metabolism shifts to a different mechanism for producing energy to keep your organ systems functioning. This mechanism involves ketosis or the breakdown of stored fats in lieu of your daily dietary intake. Ketosis along with an individual's propensity for sweating while sleeping can produce strong odors that are noticeable upon awakening. The staleness of these odors can be removed while sleeping if you crack a window or use a fan with an open bedroom door.

Leaving the bedroom window open will affect the temperature of the room, which is a major consideration for virtually all sleepers. The variability here is enormous as some people sleep more comfortably when the thermometer measures *below* 60 degrees Fahrenheit whereas others prefer 70 degrees or *above*. Scientific studies have not been able to prove conclusively that there is an ideal sleeping temperature although research does lean in support of a cooler environment. However, this information adds little to *your* sleep if you have developed a preference for a warmer environment.

If your insomnia is exacerbated by a painful condition such as arthritis or low back problems, then a cooler environment could make that worse. Moreover, many insomniacs suffer from a type of physical tenseness that produces vasoconstriction (tightening) of the blood vessels in the skin. This reduces blood flow and creates a feeling of chilliness in the insomniac. As such, when going to bed, the insomniac already feels cool and may require additional blankets. In all these situations, lowering the room temperature is more likely to lead to discomfort. Finding the right combination with fresh air, appropriate blankets and a quiet fan must take into account your personal preferences.

If, however, you sleep in the same room with someone else who has different fresh air and temperature requirements, you may need to be more adaptable. If the environment feels too cold, then a hot shower before bedtime can work magic. Or, if the room is too hot, a lukewarm bath or shower can dissipate some of the heat off of your body surface to cool you down. Again, the use of blankets and a quiet fan for your side of the bed can also make a difference.

15

EAT RIGHT, SLEEP RIGHT

QUICK GUIDE

Problem: Your diet affects your sleep.

Cause: Heavy meals at bedtime promoting indigestion and poor diets in general will lead to poor health and bad sleep.

Solution: Never eat a large meal close to bedtime and re-evaluate your food intake to insure lots of fruits, vegetables and whole grains — the foundation of any good diet.

◆ ◆ ◆

When you awaken in the morning, there are a number of situations and activities that will occur throughout the day that will affect the next night's rest. As we've mentioned, getting up and out of bed fairly quickly is a prime factor in teaching you to mentally and physically separate your sleep from your waking periods.

There are many other daytime and evening factors that also enhance or limit your capacity for sleep, including your diet, mealtimes, use of alcohol, cigarettes and caffeine, your sexual and exercise habits, your propensity for napping, and finally your style of handling worries and stress throughout the day.

A healthy diet has a very positive influence on your sleep, just as an unhealthy diet has a negative one. A healthy diet for most people consists of a lot of fruits and vegetables along with a variety of whole grains and selected dairy products and animal proteins. A balanced diet of this sort provides a solid nutritional base for your body's metabolism that, in turn, adds to your ability to remain fit and healthy.

Conversely, there is little question that a poor or unbalanced diet can lead to poorer health, perhaps more infections such as colds or flu, or more aches and pains from muscle strains and so forth. At the most fundamental level, then, if your diet is poor and your health suffers, you can expect any number of minor ailments to interfere with your sleep, whether it's a cold that interferes with your breathing, a backache that awakens you when you roll over in bed or indigestion that prevents the onset of sleep.

Eating at regular times may also aid your sleep on two counts. First, it promotes consistency that may keep you in synch with your natural biological rhythm. Second, if you maintain a schedule for your last meal of the day at a time that's not too late in the evening, then your digestion is less likely to interfere with your sleep. Large or heavy meals eaten within a couple of hours from bedtime may promote a variety of gastric distresses throughout the night, notably esophageal reflux where the digestive juices back up from the stomach into the esophagus to cause heartburn.

You may also be able to use specific foods in a targeted manner to promote better sleep. Foods that are higher in L-tryptophan may aid some people's slumber although the scientific evidence for this remains incomplete. Still, many insomniacs report some success with a turkey and cheese sandwich as a late evening snack. Other sources of naturally occurring L-tryptophan can be considered as well, but the supplement version remains off the market since the contamination problems of a few years back.

Whether or not other supplements, including melatonin, have a role in improving sleep remains unproven albeit many nutrition-oriented stores would be delighted to have you believe otherwise. On the other hand, if you have an investigative type of mind, enjoy perusing health magazines, and feel comfortable taking nutritional supplements, it may be reasonable to pursue such a path. While certain benefits have yet to be clearly proven regarding supplemental vitamins and other nutrients, it is also clear that scientific research into these areas is very limited. Therefore, the medical-scientific community may be uninformed, perhaps even misguided, about alternative approaches to some health issues.

It is of course at your own risk that you choose to experiment with supplements that may cause unknown and potentially dangerous side-effects, but supposedly we live in a free society where the individual is permitted to explore this path.

16

ALCOHOL, CAFFEINE AND NICOTINE

QUICK GUIDE

Problem: Your use of alcohol, caffeine and nicotine are interfering with your sleep.

Cause: All three substances can interfere with either your ability to fall asleep or stay asleep by producing mini-withdrawal states.

Solution: Reduce or refrain from using these drugs altogether or at least after dinner. Caffeine may require an earlier stopping time; nicotine may permit a later one.

Alcohol, nicotine and caffeine ought to be a proverbial no-brainer when it comes to sleep, yet these drugs are so commonplace that it is more unusual than not to meet someone who doesn't use any of them. Moreover, there are many people who use these drugs and sleep fine; therefore, the real issue is how might each of these substances affect an insomniac.

Nicotine has the most subtle impact by affecting your breathing over time. In the short run, if you smoke close to bedtime, you may temporarily stimulate yourself, then experience a mild nicotine withdrawal state throughout the night. In this withdrawal, the body craves another dose of nicotine, but must wait until the morning to receive it. This could lead to restless sleep and some awakenings.

Alcohol's impact is more insidious than nicotine because it can actually sedate you and promote deep sleep in the early portion of your slumber. But, like nicotine, when the alcohol wears off by the middle of the night or earlier, a mini-withdrawal state occurs that yields a definite lightening of your sleep. In other words, while alcohol could help to induce sleep, it will create difficulties in remaining asleep. It is not uncommon for someone who drinks near bedtime to arouse in the middle of the night and not be able to return to sleep.

Caffeine acts as a stimulant and a highly effective one in a variety of situations. Its use close to bedtime can produce a very attentive state that will be an obstacle to falling asleep. Caffeine is usually served in four categories of beverages and food: coffee, tea, sodas and chocolate. The amount of caffeine varies in each of these items, but all of them can have sufficient levels to disturb sleep. Once again, a mini-withdrawal state can occur in the middle of the night if you are a chronic caffeine user.

While it would be easy to recommend stopping the use of alcohol, cigarettes and caffeine to promote your overall health, for the purpose of improving your sleep, I would only suggest that you consider limiting the use of these substances. In particular, reducing or eliminating entirely any of these agents after dinner time could prove a simple remedy for some insomniacs. Making such a commitment will also facilitate your ability to cease using these drugs at a later date if you so desire.

17

SEX AND EXERCISE

QUICK GUIDE

Problem: Exercise is not helping your sleep.

Cause: If you engage in exercise too late in the day, its alerting influence may last beyond your normal bedtime.

Solution: Light exercise, such as walking in the evening is fine, but heavier exertion should be reserved for earlier in the day and preferably before dinner.

◆ ◆ ◆

Physical activity can have a dramatic influence on your sleep propensity. You may remember a time at a younger age when vigorous physical exertion during the daytime led to solid sleep at night.

In point of fact, the average person would benefit tremendously by engaging in significant physical exercise every day, and for a time frame probably much longer than is generally prescribed. It is not a question of gaining some aerobic capacity effect (e.g. running) or engaging in extended moderate activity (e.g. walking) although either of these exercises may provide healthy results.

The real issue with respect to sleep is that physical activity is a natural part of being human. To think otherwise goes against the grain of virtually all of human history except for the last few sedentary decades of the twentieth century. People are built to do things, whether it's walking, bicycling, traipsing up and down steps, jogging to the corner market and so on.

In modern times, this is why extended activities like hiking, endurance swimming, long walks, or even golf (no electric carts, please) encourage you to use your body over a period of time that in many ways more closely matches what your level of activity might have been years ago no matter where you lived. Perhaps one day our society will evolve to recapture this lost emphasis on physicality. If so, the norm will be to engage in physical activities throughout various portions of the day, some perhaps related to work, others to play.

Nowadays, however, exercise often gets blocked off into predetermined segments of your life. You may jog in the morning, or walk in the evening. Certainly this is better than nothing, but because you become accustomed to only one portion of the day to exert yourself, the timing of this exercise may produce an undesirable outcome. For example, if you run aerobically or lift weights later in the evening, say a few hours before bedtime, the aftereffect may actually alert you and inhibit your ability to fall asleep. Conversely, if you exercise late in the afternoon before dinner, the immediate overheating of your body through physical exertion may promote a steeper decline of your body temperature as you approach bedtime and thus promote your ability to fall asleep.

In summary, some exercise is better than none, but timing may prove pivotal in determining the response. Such is the case with sexual activity, too, of which almost nothing is written about with regards to sleep.

I have emphasized the use of the bedroom only for sleep, but this was not meant to preclude or hamper your sex life in anyway. In fact, in terms of the concept of associations about which most of sleep hygiene is predicated upon, sex and sleep are inextricably linked. After all, most sexual encounters for the vast majority of individuals occur at night, in bed and just prior to sleep. The second most common encounter would probably be in the morning, in bed, and waking up from sleep.

Your sex life, therefore, affects your sleep life. Unfortunately, very little research is available to suggest what the impact might be. Moreover, in discussing this with different people you will discover a surprising range of responses. For example, some people note that sex, or orgasm in particular, will always help them to fall asleep, while others will declare the exact opposite, that is, sex will alert them so much that they cannot fall asleep. This range of opinions occurs in both men and women.

Thus, responses to both exercise and sex can be different for different people, yet there is no question that our bodies were made both to engage in physical activity and love-making. Interestingly, both experiences can lead to considerable reduction in physical tension. This tension by the way is believed to be one of the leading physical components of insomnia for many people.

Sometimes the phrase, "somatized tension" is used to describe this problem. These words mean that a series of thoughts, feelings, sensations, really everything that makes one human, may fester in the body in the form of tension energy instead of finding an appropriate release.

Learning to appreciate how exercise and sex can reduce some of this tension energy may prove useful in treating your insomnia.

18

MAKE NAPS SHORT AND EARLY

QUICK GUIDE

Problem: Napping during the day comes easy, yet it seems to be affecting nighttime sleep.

Cause: Naps that are too long or too late in the day will reduce your overall sleep pressure and thus cause problems at night.

Solution: Napping is fine if you accept that you only need so much sleep every 24-hour period. Limit your nap to earlier in the day and no more than thirty minutes, if not less.

◆ ◆ ◆

The question of napping is raised by some insomniacs who are often puzzled by their ability to fall asleep during the daytime on some occasions, yet continue to have difficulty falling asleep at night. There is nothing fundamentally wrong with napping, but it is important to appreciate and follow a few guidelines if you choose to nap so that it will not interfere with your nighttime sleep.

Foremost, assume that in the course of any 24-hour period you will need only so much sleep — it could be eight hours or it might only be six. If you choose to use up some of your sleep time during the day, that's all right, particularly if you feel refreshed after a nap, and it doesn't interfere with your nighttime sleep.

Naps may interfere with your night time sleep in several ways. First, if you nap too late in the afternoon or early in the evening, your mind and body are not likely to be in the mood to fall asleep again at night. Second, if you nap for a long period, for example, beyond one hour (for some beyond 20 minutes), this can produce a similar problem; namely, your mind and body will have already experienced a sufficient period of sleep so as to not feel ready to engage in sleep again for several more hours.

So, the later or the longer you nap, there is more potential for this behavior to become self-defeating with respect to your nighttime efforts. In short, you may find yourself staying up well beyond midnight before genuine sleepiness reappears to lead you naturally toward a good night's slumber.

Why nap at all then?

Harvey Penick, the famous golf instructor was fond of saying, "if I ask you to take an aspirin, don't take the whole bottle." The same goes for napping. If you use a very brief catnap early rather than later in the day to refresh you, it's doubtful that such a short sleep period will interfere with your nighttime sleep. In fact, some sleep specialists believe that your ability to nap in such a manner will build confidence in your overall ability to fall asleep and thus enhance your attempt at night.

Moreover, it must be pointed out that napping is common in many cultures; often, a lengthy nap period at midday and a shorter nighttime sleep period are the norm. One reason for splitting your sleep into two distinct time periods may be explained by our natural biological clock — the circadian rhythm. As mentioned, at night the circadian rhythm induces our body temperature to decrease, which promotes falling and staying asleep. A similar temperature drop may occur during the daytime for a much briefer time span. Around or just after lunchtime, the body's temperature begins to level off or briefly decline. This time period can last for a few minutes to a few hours, but some degree of sleepiness is produced in virtually everyone. Caffeine can of course mask this reflex; but notwithstanding the use of stimulants like coffee, almost anyone could easily adopt a system that promotes napping or *siesta* in synchrony with this short, natural change in body temperature. This should be coupled however with an expectation for a shorter nighttime sleep period. Then again, such a schedule must realistically fit in with your work and home life so that the benefit of a short nap clearly outweighs any disadvantages, inconveniences or conflicts.

As you can see, there are reasons why it may be easier to feel sleepy during the day and to actually nod off for several minutes or even a couple of hours; however, I must reiterate that you probably need only so much sleep in the course of any 24-hour period. If you sleep too much during the day, then you remove or reduce your natural physiological sleep pressure that could have served you well that night. Remember, *sleep pressure builds to higher levels the longer you remain awake* unless you suffer from a psychiatric illness such as manic-depression in which shortened sleep length can trigger a manic episode. Generally, lengthy naps are likely to diminish sleep pressure and cause more difficulty when attempting to fall asleep at night.

Last, it is also helpful to recognize the basic psychology of being able to fall asleep during the day. The feeling of sleepiness can sometimes occur as a response to a boring or difficult emotional situation. If you have trouble falling asleep at night, but notice a much easier propensity for doing so during the day, it may be worthwhile to examine if there are specific situations that produce this response. If for example you must attend a boring lecture or class or meeting in the early afternoon, you may notice that it's relatively easy to fall asleep.

True boredom is a wonderful thing if your goal is to fall asleep. Many an insomniac wishes that she could recreate a genuine boring state around bedtime because the chances for falling asleep would be so much higher. This is why some sleep doctors preach that it is necessary to avoid all types of stimulation close to bedtime. This may refer to what you're watching on TV or listening to on the radio, or what you may be reading, but of equal if not greater importance, it refers to how you might be stimulating your mind and body through conversation and other interpersonal encounters with friends and family.

With respect to more disturbing emotions, there is no question that some people attempt to escape from unpleasant feelings by becoming sleepy and/or falling asleep. In some respects, this can be quite healthy, particularly for your nighttime sleep as it may give you a necessary breather from emotional turmoil that might sort itself out with a good night's rest, maybe even through the wonders of dreaming.

With respect to napping, however, if you discover that your sleepy feeling is preceded by some problematic emotional conflict, you may gain some sleep, but perhaps you are merely postponing your need to confront your feelings more directly. If so, we might expect that even though you had little difficulty falling asleep after lunch, you would in all probability not have such an easy time of it at bedtime, particularly as you may have compounded the problem by having used up your natural sleep pressure with a daytime nap.

To nap or not to nap then can have subtle wrinkles that must be carefully ironed out so that it is clear to you why and how short sleep periods may be beneficial or harmful to your nighttime sleep.

Now let's return to more general questions about how emotions, stress, and managing one's feelings have an effect on your sleep. We've mentioned a few points here in relationship to napping, which has served as a useful starting point. We'll delve a bit deeper to see how your mood and your emotions can have a dramatic impact on your complete sleep cycle.

19

STOP WORRYING AND START SLEEPING

QUICK GUIDE

Problem: Mental attitudes and emotional worries are disrupting your sleep.

Cause: Worries and other negative emotions produce negative mental associations that keep you awake in bed thinking about your problems.

Solution: Consider a short worry session earlier in the day to focus on your conflicts at a time unrelated to sleep. Also consider the help of a friend or perhaps a mental health professional who can teach you successful psychological coping skills to improve the way you handle stress.

◆ ◆ ◆

Your mental attitude prior to bedtime has a great — perhaps the greatest — influence on your capacity to sleep soundly. This attitude actually may encompass a number of aspects including your state of relaxation, tension in your body, anxieties and worries, and your overall mental health.

Mental health is an on-going process filtering into every aspect of your life. For example, tension in the body does not suddenly arise a few minutes before bedtime; rather, it usually builds throughout the day and may eventually cause an inability to relax sufficiently to fall asleep.

Dealing with mental health issues is not something to put off. Learning to recognize tension in the body and learning how to relax can be worked on throughout the day. Meditation, yoga, deep breathing, imagery work, and light physical exercise are a few techniques that can help you relax. It may prove especially helpful to engage in some relaxing behavior in the evening as you wind down toward bedtime.

Physical tension or the inability to relax may stem from unresolved emotional conflicts or problems. People who have difficulty sleeping may discover that the source of their tension is pent-up feelings such as fear, sadness, guilt, anger or frustration. Others may notice more ill-defined feelings such as anxiety.

Learning to recognize these emotions is a necessary first step in improving your mental health. The more these feelings are avoided, denied or suppressed, the more likely they will boil over onto the surface. A prime example could be someone suffering from insomnia, who doesn't realize that his or her inability to fall asleep is a red flag signaling emotional distress. The longer you avoid the warning, the more likely the insomnia will continue, if not worsen. And, sometimes, the insomnia will turn out to be a harbinger of depression, which may develop more than a year after the start of the insomnia.

The single most consistently destructive emotional state that affects our sleep revolves around anticipated problems: in short, our worries. Worrying about the future is one of the surest paths to insomnia! On a rational level, it is of some benefit to realize that: **it is rare for a state of worry to solve the problem that is being worried about.**

If you allow yourself to appreciate that worries only beget more worries, you may want to explore what some call "worry sessions." At a point earlier in the day (no later than after dinner), some people have found it useful to focus their anxieties into a single short session (through self-talk or pad and paper) with the understanding that once the time period (say, ten to twenty minutes) is completed, no further worrying is permitted. Specifically, a commitment is made to avoid being held hostage by fretful thoughts. While such an approach may be appealing, some people's anxieties may get the best of them and simply initiate a cascading process that knows no end.

It is certainly natural and common to experience some anxiety during the day; however, the feeling of anxiety is often a mask for another even stronger emotion that may be more threatening than so-called worrying. For example, if you are having a problem at work such that you are very *angry* with your boss while at the same time you are *fearful* of losing your job if you were to express that anger, the mind's natural defenses have a way of prevailing so that you instead believe your problem is that you are nervous about something that is supposedly ill-defined.

Why would this be so? Simply, if you believed that you were accurate in your perception of the threat, that is, your boss would dismiss you if you expressed your genuine anger, then in many real-life circumstances, the better part of valor would often be to bite your tongue. Anxiety is sure to follow in such situations unless you develop the skill of learning to recognize and appreciate the depths of your anger and fear without having to act on them in a way that might jeopardize your job.

Some people's emotional distress requires professional help. A poor sleeper may develop the belief that if she could only sleep better, then her bad feelings would disappear. In fact, many people feel they are depressed because of poor sleep. This may be accurate, but it is more likely a two-way street: depression may induce poor sleep, while poor sleep might worsen depression.

The relationship between mental health and sleep is not always straightforward. Talking with your physician, a mental health professional, a clergyman or a close friend about emotional problems may be one of the most successful strategies you can use to improve your sleep. If your particular style of handling worries and stress is a major contributor to your sleeplessness, then a mental health professional, in just a few short sessions, may be able to teach you a different coping style that will also improve your problems with insomnia.

20

BEYOND SLEEP HYGIENE

QUICK GUIDE

Problem: Sleep hygiene has helped to reduce but not eliminate your problems with insomnia.

Cause: There are many different types of insomnia, all of which benefit from the applications of sleep hygiene, but some of which require additional measures.

Solution: Consider seeking help from a sleep specialist to help you uncover physical sleep disorders that might be a deeper cause for your sleeplessness.

Sleep ought to be a natural process occurring without significant effort. **You let yourself fall asleep.**

Why a person loses this natural ability is often related to many, if not most of the items we've addressed in our focus on sleep hygiene. Sleep hygiene is a simple set of guidelines that will help you to appreciate what was hopefully at one point in your life a very natural process. By following these guidelines you give yourself the opportunity to recapture the natural feeling that enhanced your ability to fall asleep and stay asleep. Moreover, sleep hygiene guidelines provide you with some flexibility and allow for individual adaptation to your personal needs. Incorporating these principles into your waking and sleeping habits is often a simple and effective way to improve your sleep.

But now the question may arise: what if sleep hygiene turns out to be only half the picture?

Sleep Hygiene, the first installment of the *INSOMNIA CURES* series was written for the vast majority of mild to moderate insomniacs whose difficulties will usually respond to the straightforward cognitive-behavioral changes suggested through the principles and practice of sleep hygiene. Even among those who have more complex forms of insomnia, sleep hygiene will almost always offer some hope and yield some improvement.

But some patients with complex insomnia may need more help. They may for example require the services of a sleep specialist to guide them through more exacting strategies such as sleep restriction therapy coupled with the use of extensive diary and journal exercises. In such instances, working with a professional trained in the subtleties and nuances of sleep medicine can enhance your level of success.

For those of you who have persisting difficulties, I would like to leave you with two important considerations to guide you in your further quest of a cure.

First, it is imperative to recognize that insomnia is often a problem caused by several things, not just one thing; yet, like a jigsaw puzzle, you must start with one piece. As you join more pieces of that puzzle together, a picture begins to form. However, it can prove frustrating and overwhelming if you are routinely selecting a part to the puzzle that doesn't fit. Where to start your attack on the problem of sleeplessness can prove crucial to your success, for when you discover a key piece to your personal insomnia puzzle, many of the other parts will fall naturally into place. It is for these reasons that sleep hygiene often, but not always, proves to be the very best program with which to initiate your exploration of your insomnia problem. Soon thereafter, other factors may be taken into consideration. And, in most cases, learning about one or two different approaches to insomnia will be sufficient to cure your problem. Usually you will not need to learn about all the causes of insomnia, nor will you have to experiment with all the different types of treatment plans. One or two approaches will work fine, just as laying your fingers on a few key pieces of a puzzle will help you forge ahead in your discovery of the whole picture.

As indicated in the Preface and to close out this book, let me make it clear, once again, that while sleep hygiene may be the very best first step to take in this process, it may not yield a cure. In my personal and professional experience, I have learned that many insomniacs, contrary to the current and prevailing scientific view from the field of sleep medicine, actually suffer from very subtle sleep breathing and sleep movement disorders. These disorders are not easy to diagnose because the current technology used to evaluate sleep is similar to the situation in which one would find oneself using a magnifying glass to search for something that can only be observed with a microscope. New technology is emerging every year and soon, I predict, it will become clearer to our field of medicine, that physical factors or disorders are really a much greater contributor to insomnia than has been previously recognized.

The wonderful thing about this is that such technology will ultimately confirm what most doctors were taught and hopefully are still taught in medical school: **that the patient in some way or another always carries a special knowledge and understanding of their own problem.** Although this knowledge may not be particularly scientific, it still provides explanations that physicians and scientists should never forget to acknowledge *and* utilize for the patient's benefit. In the instance of sleep problems, patients have long offered the following refrain: "doctor, if I could just sleep better, I'm sure my depression would improve." To this refrain, many patients receive an equally resounding chorus from their doctors that goes something like this: "actually, if we just treated your depression, I bet your sleep problems would get better, too." Both doctor and patient are probably on the right track, but I predict with the advent of greater technological sophistication, we will learn that the treatment of subtle sleep breathing and sleep movement disorders will cure a much larger number of insomniacs than most sleep specialists, let alone doctors, would have expected based on our current understanding of sleep medicine.

I offer this last bit of speculation for those of you who feel particularly frustrated in your quest for better sleep and feel that in some ways your anguished cries for help have fallen on ears deafened by what appears to be "a wax build-up" of modern medicine. In time, I trust that for many of you, a closer inspection of these subtle sleep problems will remove the last remaining obstacles in your journey down the path to healthy sleep.

Good luck and sweet dreams!

EPILOGUE

At the beginning of the 21st century, the field of sleep medicine must still be considered a relatively new, if not primitive field. We still know very little about the fundamental ways in which sleeping or dreaming affect our lives and health. We know that sleep and dreams are important, but our ability to define and describe normal sleep and dreaming remains remarkably limited.

Insomnia is a sleep disorder of which a great deal of descriptive information has been gathered, but there is only a small amount of knowledge on the underlying mechanisms that cause or promote insomnia. Currently, there is a great deal of emphasis on the behavioral or psycho-physiological explanations for insomnia, which implicate one's attitude, beliefs, habits, and circumstances and possibly biological predisposition as causative factors. This book has therefore focused on cognitive-behavioral treatments (CBT) for insomnia, and CBT will sometimes prove curative for some insomniacs and quite helpful to others. Still, it is interesting and puzzling that the field of sleep medicine has not been able to develop a definitive program that *consistently* and *completely* cures insomnia, particularly for those with more severe sleep complaints.

In my opinion, sleep medicine has failed to make greater strides in the treatment of insomnia because it has tended to narrowly focus on two prevailing approaches to the problem. The first, as described, is the cognitive-behavioral method, which is often very helpful but typically not curative. The second is pharmacotherapy, that is, treatment with sedatives or anxiety-reducing drugs or antidepressants. Once again, whereas these therapies may be effective in some patients, they are rarely curative except in short-term cases, and they produce adverse effects. These adverse effects are not inconsequential and may include higher mortality rates among those who use sedatives on a nightly basis. And, as of June, 2001, there has only been one published double-blind, placebo-controlled study of antidepressants in the treatment of primary insomnia (insomnia without some other medical or psychiatric cause), and although the results were statistically significant, the actual improvement, from the patient's perspective, was described as "light to moderate."

What then are the obstacles that might be preventing the field of sleep medicine from maximizing the therapeutic effects of insomnia treatments?

I believe the biggest obstacle is that sleep clinicians and researchers are unable to reconcile complaints of insomnia with some physical abnormality in the patient. In other words, insomnia appears to be a problem in the patient's mind, therefore, how are we going to help the patient if we cannot "see" what's actually malfunctioning. Because of this mindset, physicians and therapists and others who treat patients with insomnia complaints automatically assume that when the patient says, "there is something wrong with my sleep" or "I don't sleep very well," it must mean that something is wrong with the patient's mental functioning, which then is deemed to be the cause of the problem. On the other hand, if I show up in the Emergency Department complaining that my arm hurts and the x-ray says it's broken, it is much easier to see cause and effect and therefore much easier to treat.

This psychological mindset, in my opinion, represents the largest obstacle blocking the path toward greater advances in the treatment of insomnia. When patients say something is wrong with their sleep, then I accept that something is wrong with their sleep. My task as a clinician and researcher is to find out what that something is. So, I start, as discussed in this book, with the concept of sleep quality, which regrettably, many practitioners avoid discussing or considering when managing their insomnia patients. And, like those patients who commonly confuse sleep quantity with the concept of quality, many doctors and therapists have become accustomed to thinking about correcting sleep quantity complaints with drugs or psychotherapy or cognitive-behavioral therapy. In our experience, however, even if insomnia improves with these methods, a sleep quality problem may persist, particularly in those who have had sleep problems for years or who would describe their insomnia as moderate or severe.

Because we have invariably asked insomniacs about the quality of their sleep and have probed this area in great depth, we have been fortunate to uncover a very surprising connection between insomnia and a physical sleep disorder, commonly called sleep apnea—now designated as sleep-disordered breathing or SDB for short. We have researched insomnia in several types of patients. For example, we have conducted research studies on women who suffered rape and childhood sexual abuse; we've studied evacuees following a natural disaster; and we've worked with many adults who experienced various types of criminal victimization. In addition, I have also worked in commercial sleep clinics where many insomniacs come for treatment. In all these settings, we have been surprised to learn that the majority of insomniacs with moderate to severe sleep complaints also suffered from sleep-disordered breathing.

Sometimes SDB takes the obvious form of sleep apnea where airflow during sleep is so obstructed it actually ceases for 10 seconds or longer. In many more instances, though, SDB has taken the form of upper airway resistance, which means that the flow of air did not stop, but it was noticeably constrained as if it were being pulled through a tube whose diameter was too small to permit a smooth flow of air. Regardless of the exact description of the breathing disruption, the important point is that individuals with either type of SDB suffer from hundreds of nocturnal brain arousals or frank awakenings all through their sleep. As such, they are not really sleeping in a consolidated manner. Instead, they are waking up and returning to sleep hundreds of times per night.

Logically, one might assume that SDB ought to be one of the first things to consider in searching for the cause of insomnia. But, this approach has not been adopted routinely for one very good reason—a large number of people with SDB never develop insomnia but instead suffer from sleepiness during the daytime and at night. In other words, robbed of their sleep through hundreds of awakenings, their response is classic sleep deprivation. They are exhausted and sleepy all day and all night long and never have any difficulty going or returning to sleep. Because this fits the classic definition of sleep apnea, most physicians have become accustomed to thinking that a patient *without* sleepiness cannot have sleep-disordered breathing.

We predict that there is a different and very large group of patients who suffer these SDB-induced awakenings, but they develop insomnia instead of daytime sleepiness. We make this prediction because we have already documented rates of SDB between 50 and 90% in our research participants who enrolled in our programs for the treatment of insomnia, and we have consistently observed this diagnosis in more than 75% of insomniacs presenting to our sleep clinics.

To reiterate, *why* these awakenings promote insomnia in one person and sleepiness in another is an extremely interesting question to be researched in the future, but more importantly, our curiosity has been further piqued by having cured insomnia in patients treated for sleep-disordered breathing. SDB treatment is not as easy as taking a pill, and it may even appear threatening to some insomniacs. Nonetheless, we have worked with hundreds of research and clinic patients whose insomnia was markedly reduced or completely eliminated by successful application of SDB treatment.

Most of these patients learned how to use a breathing mask that provides continuous positive airway pressure that keeps the diameter of your "breathing tube" wide open during the night. It eliminates snoring or any other subtle breathing disruption, such as upper airway resistance, and in so doing, it eliminates the hundreds of brain arousals and awakenings throughout the night.

For these patients, it appears that fixing the sleep breathing problem was the direct path to fixing the sleep quality problem. Once sleep quality was enhanced, many of these patients reported that their insomnia was cured.

We have observed similar results in patients using special dental devices known as oral appliances. These devices stabilize the position of the jaw to maintain the diameter of your "breathing tube," and the result once again was improved airflow, decreased arousals and greatly enhanced sleep quality. In a few cases, where individuals could not tolerate the breathing mask or dental device, they proceeded to surgical interventions aimed at reducing excess tissue in the airway or stabilizing certain muscles that influence airway diameter. These patients also reported marked improvements or cures in their sleep complaints.

Still, this path may not be for every insomniac; and we have worked with many who have been unwilling to pursue this treatment even though they were clearly diagnosed with sleep-disordered breathing.

Thomas Paine said, "Time makes more converts than reason." And, in my professional clinical and research experience, I appreciate that it will take a considerable period of time for both patients, doctors and therapists to recognize that physical sleep disorders play an important role in causing or worsening insomnia. My objective as a clinician and a researcher is to get the "reasons" out there, so that people will have the opportunity to judge for themselves whether or not this pathway is relevant to their problem. Perhaps more importantly, this new knowledge will assist clinicians in recognizing the importance of treating sleep-disordered breathing among people complaining of insomnia. We are writing several new research papers every year on this topic, and in time, we expect to see a few more converts.

ENDNOTES

QUICK GUIDE

If you are considering the possibility that sleep-disordered breathing may underlie your insomnia problems, please consider these steps in pursuing such an evaluation.

Self-assessment

Spend time reading about sleep-disordered breathing so that you will be able to communicate easily with healthcare providers who, ironically, will likely know less than you do about SDB. In particular, if you do *not* snore, then it's important to read about upper airway resistance syndrome (UARS) as this could occur in people who do not snore. Again, most healthcare providers do not know much about UARS. Overall, it is in your best interest to read about SDB so that you can make your own self-assessment before contacting a healthcare provider.

Contact Healthcare Provider

Unless you are independently wealthy or have an insurance program that permits direct access to specialists, I believe it will be invaluable to make contact with a primary care provider, that is, your regular doctor, to pursue treatment for SDB. Certainly, if you are in a managed care insurance program, you may be required to do so. If you can convince or persuade your primary doctor that your chances for SDB are much higher than he or she would have imagined, then you will have made a formidable ally in your attempt to get adequate assessment and treatment for SDB once you are referred to a sleep specialist.

Sleep Specialist Contact

This will prove to be the thorniest part of the pathway because many sincere, dedicated but overworked sleep specialists have not kept abreast of the knowledge showing a relationship between insomnia and SDB. Worse, many sleep specialists are still somewhat skeptical or unaware of the advances in respiratory assessment technology to assess subtle breathing conditions such as UARS. In other words, once you get an appointment with a sleep specialist, there may still be the need to convince that doctor to conduct a sleep study on you, and you may have to request that the sleep lab be equipped with special devices known as esophageal monitors or nasal pressure transducers to adequately assess your breathing pattern. You can see how thorny this can get because it might make the doctor feel like he or she is being pushed around by someone who appears to "know too much." In my years as an internist, emergency medicine physician and sleep specialist, I've always welcomed the motivated patients who had done some "homework" before their appointments. However, I know from practical experience that the key to success in such encounters is DIPLOMACY. Sleep specialists are becoming inundated with requests for services and are being pushed by managed care pressures like all other doctors to provide faster, less comprehensive medical care. As long as you offer your self-assessment with respect and sincerity, most physicians of any type are willing to listen and consider your needs.

Treatment Options

I advise all SDB patients to try the breathing mask first because even though it might be uncomfortable and ultimately intolerable, it gives you the opportunity to experience high quality sleep almost immediately. This is worth its weight in gold because once you actually experience what happens when breathing disruption is removed from your sleep, it will greatly increase your motivation to follow through on whatever treatment approach you choose. For individuals that are fairly overweight, the breathing mask almost always appears to be the best option. For people who are normal or under weight, oral appliances are often most effective. But in each of these instances, remember that there are various types of breathing masks and pressurized air machines and various types of oral appliances. You get what you pay for, so always consider the possibility that you will need to make adjustments to the equipment you are using or the need for new, more advanced equipment if things are not improving as you think they might. In such instances, trial and error during an interval of one to several months may be needed to optimize your treatment.

Conclusion

In future books, we will talk more about treating SDB in insomniacs. New advances in SDB treatment are being published several times per year as the medical profession has come to realize that sleep-disordered breathing is incredibly common. With this new research emphasis alone, eventually more people will become aware of the possible connection between SDB and insomnia. If you seek to stay current on this topic, please look for our new research articles as well those of other researchers in this blossoming field of sleep medicine. And, every few months or so, you can also check for regular updates through our web site www.nightmaretreatment.com.

ABOUT THE AUTHOR

Barry Krakow, M.D. is a board certified internist and sleep disorders specialist. He is the medical director of the Center for Sleep Medicine & Nightmare Treatment and the Sleep & Human Health Institute. He has conducted a decade of research on the treatment of nightmares, insomnia and posttraumatic stress and has treated many sleep disorders patients and trauma survivors. Dr. Krakow is a member of the American Academy of Sleep Medicine and the Sleep Research Society, a consulting editor for the journal *Dreaming* and a reviewer for many sleep, trauma and psychiatric journals. He lives in Albuquerque, New Mexico with his wife and two children.